Bob Tells All

Sheila Hollins
Valerie Sinason

Illustrated by Beth Webb

St George's Mental Health Library
LONDON

First Published in Great Britain 1993
by St George's Mental Health Library,
Cranmer Terrace, Tooting, London SW17 0RE
Series Editor: Professor Sheila Hollins

ISBN 1 874439 03 6

British Library Cataloging - in - Publication Data

A catalogue record for this book is available from the
British Library

Typeset, printed and bound in Great Britain by
HGA Printing Company Ltd, Brentford Middlesex

The Sovereign Series: Language beyond words.
Other titles now available:
Peter's New Home
A New Home in the Community
When Dad Died
When Mum Died
Jenny Speaks Out
In preparation:
Hugging and Touching

Please photocopy the order form
on page 63 of this book, or write
for an information leaflet to:
St George's Mental Health Library
The Division of Psychiatry of Disability
St. George's Hospital Medical School,
Cranmer Terrace, London SW17 0RE
Tel: 081 672 9944 ext.55501

Dedication

To all those people with learning disabilities who have shared their experience of abuse with us.

Acknowledgements

With thanks to the following whose interest and encouragement has made this book possible:
Members of the Division of Psychiatry of Disability at St George's Hospital Medical School,
and of the Tavistock Clinic Foundation.

Bob moved to a group home.

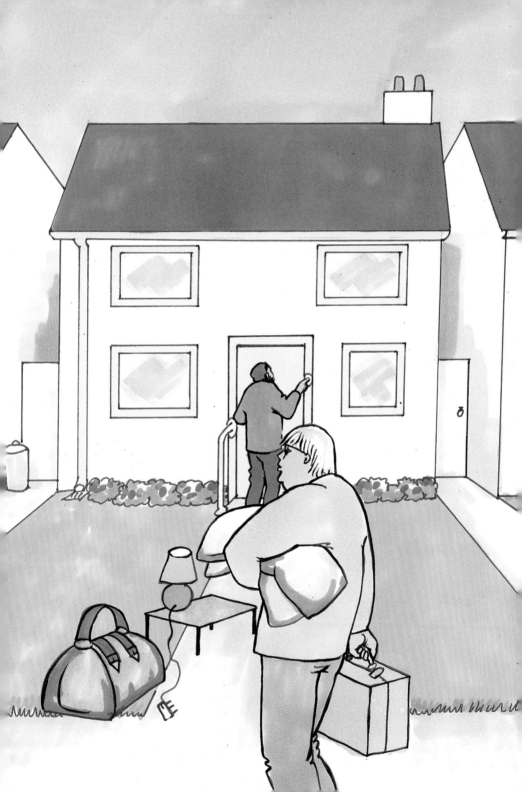

Jon helped him unpack.

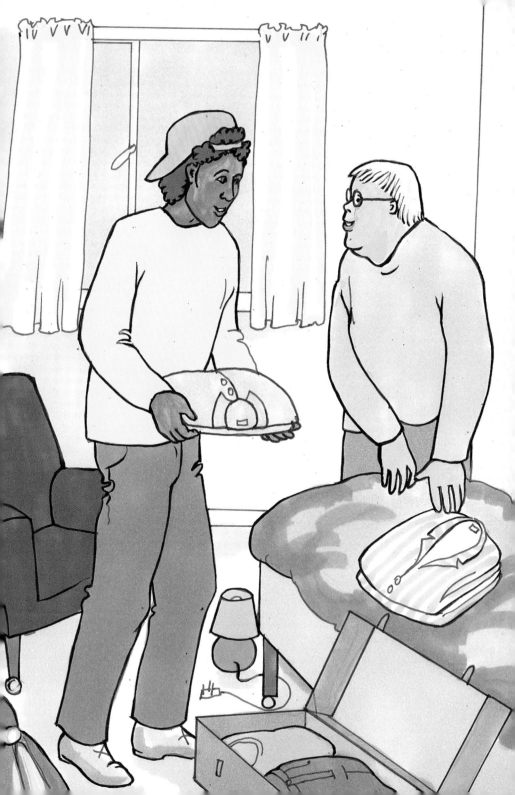

Bob liked his new friends.

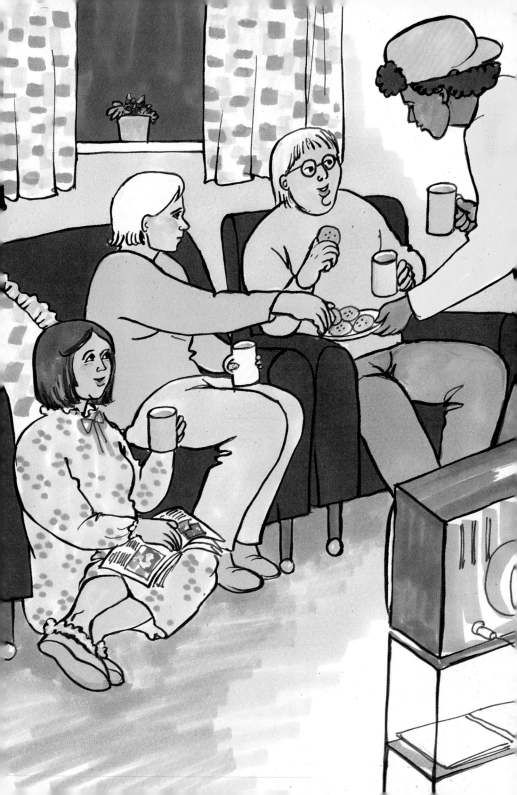

That night, Bob woke
everyone with his screaming.

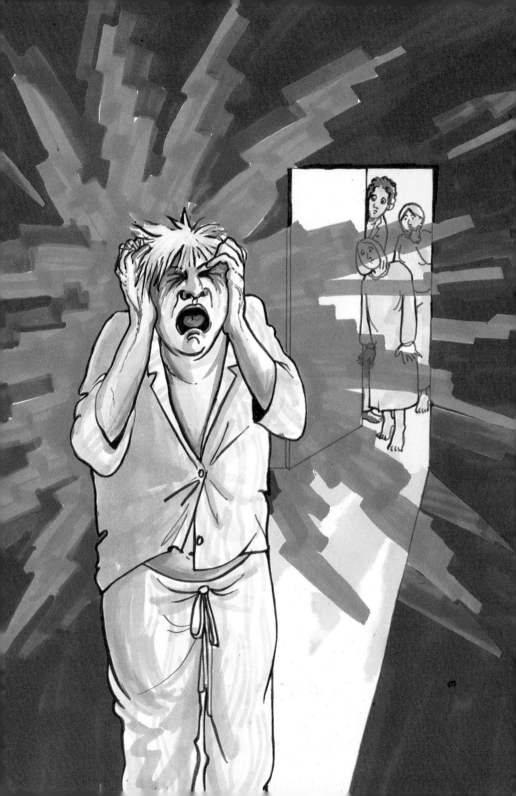

In the morning, Bob went crazy.

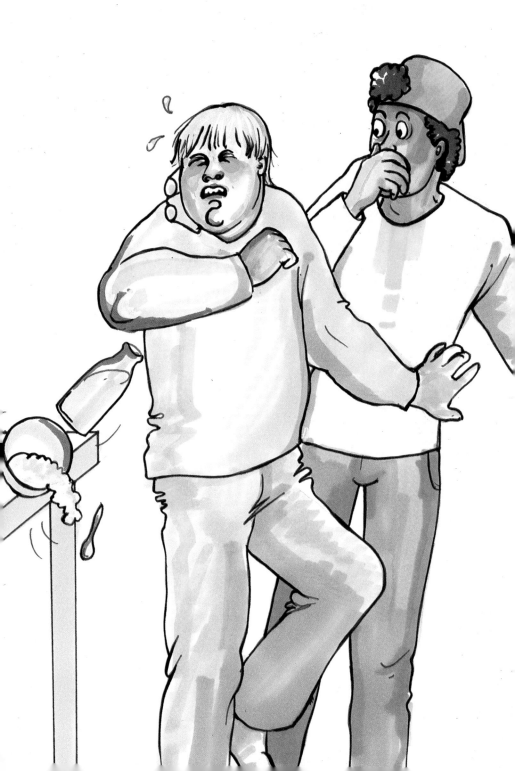

"What's wrong?" asked Jon.

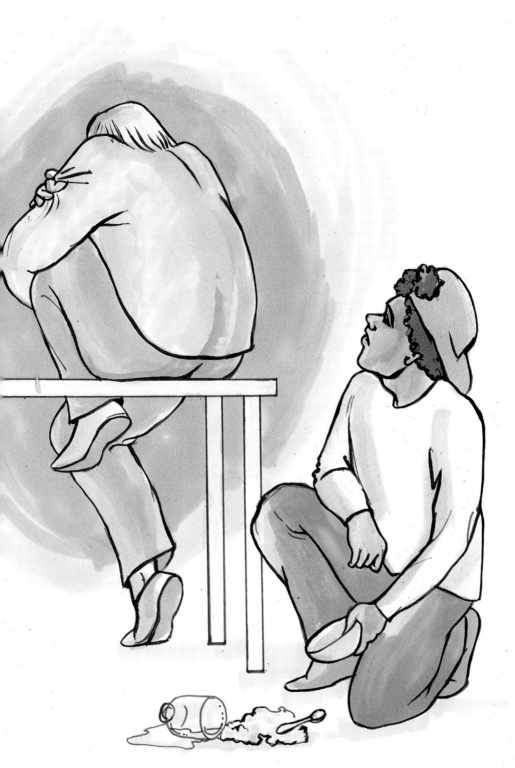

"Shut up or I'll give you one!" shouted Bob.

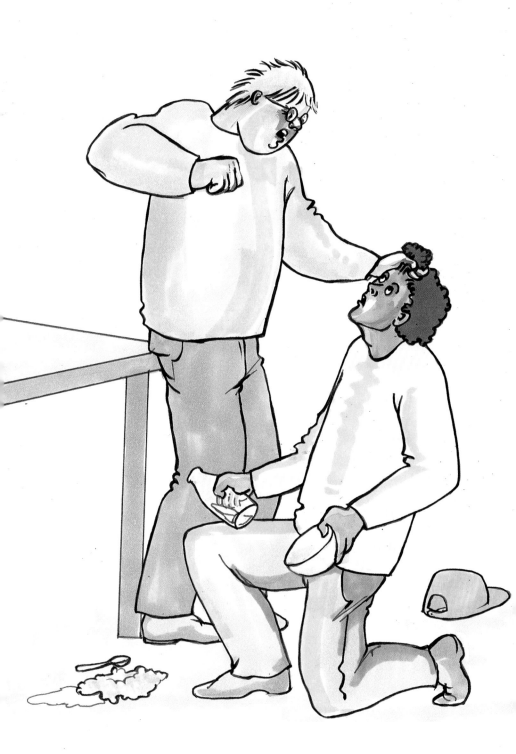

Bob smashed up his room.

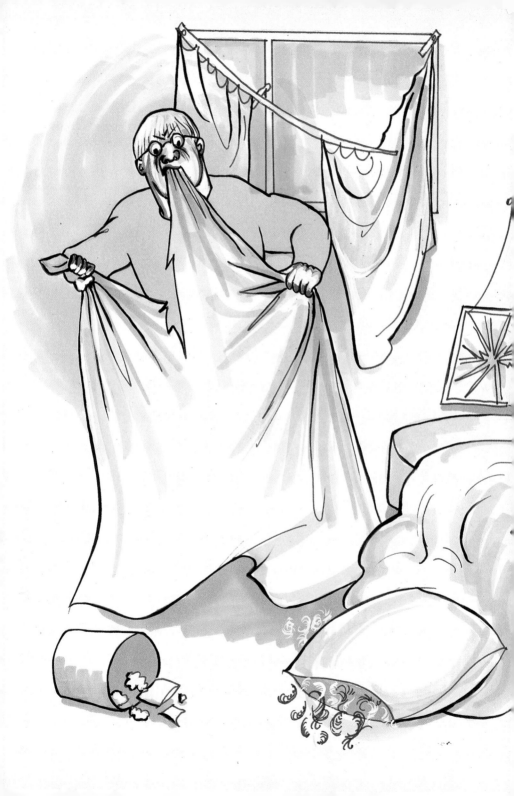

Bob felt terrible.
He didn't know what to do.

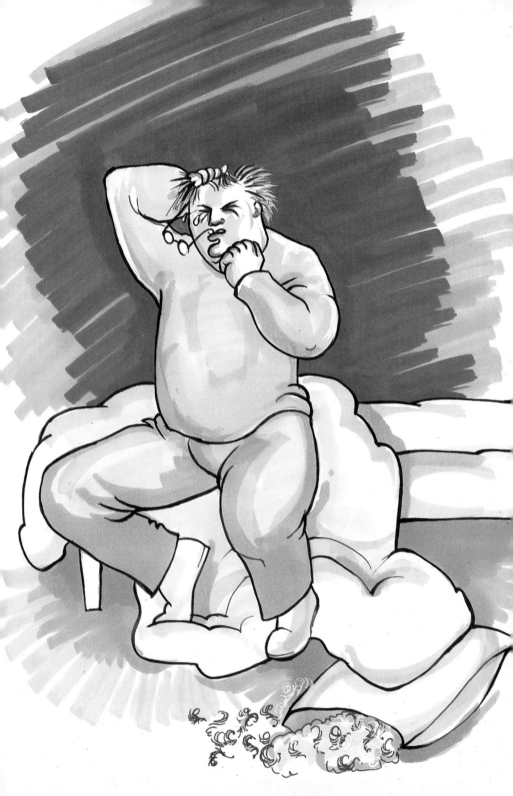

Jon rang Steve,
their social worker.
Jon said, "We're all
frightened of Bob!"

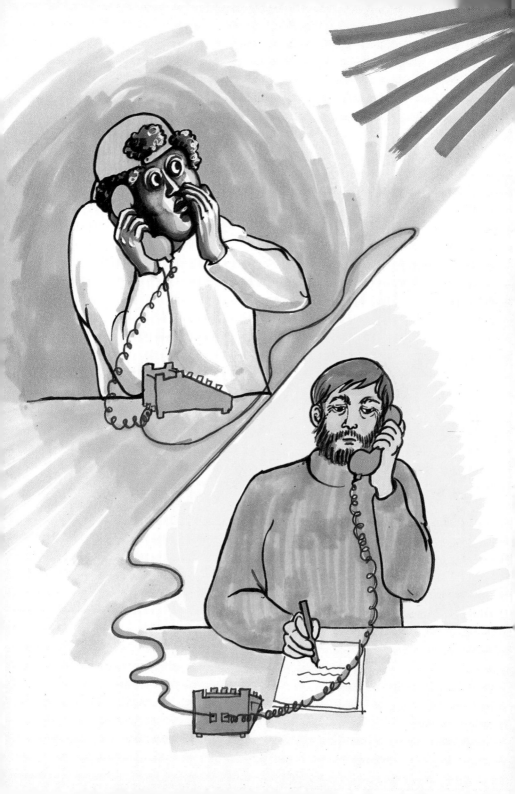

Steve came straight away.

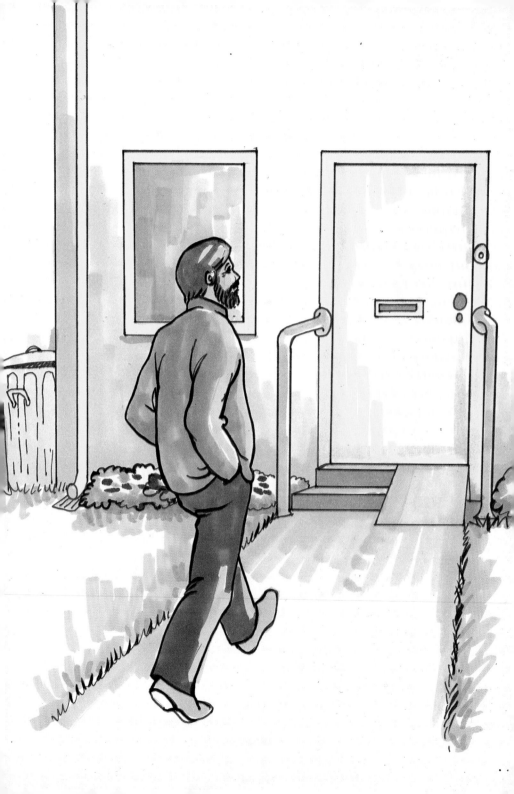

"Bob's upstairs!" said everyone.

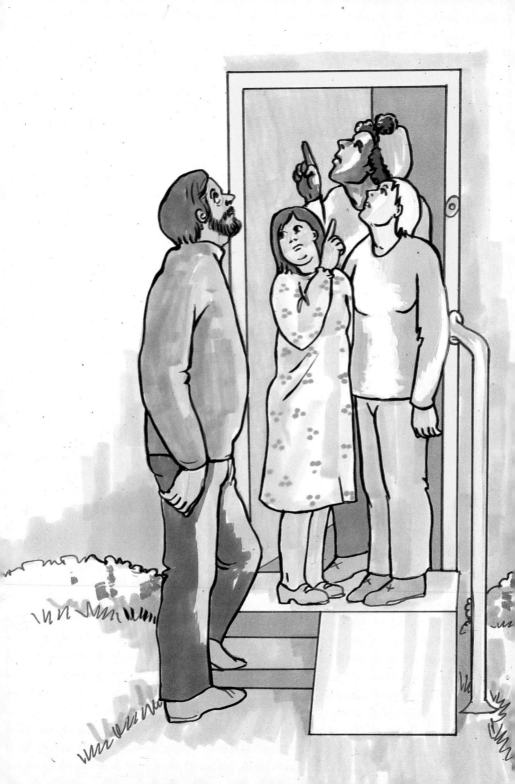

Steve knocked on Bob's door.

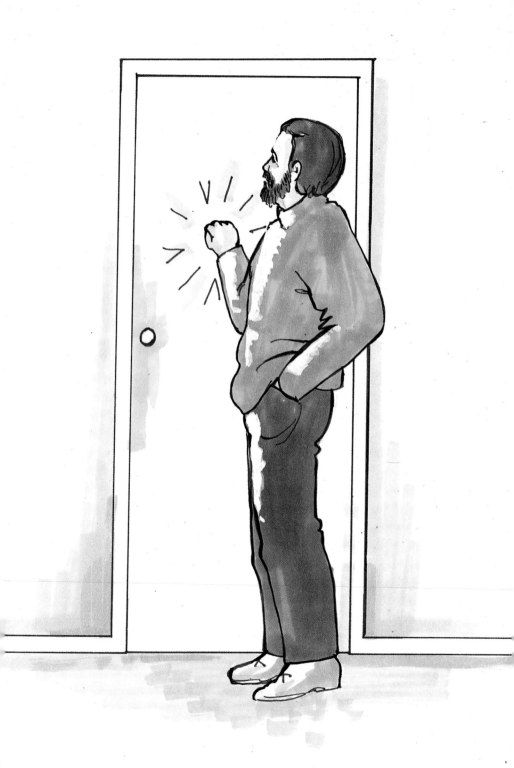

Bob was scared.

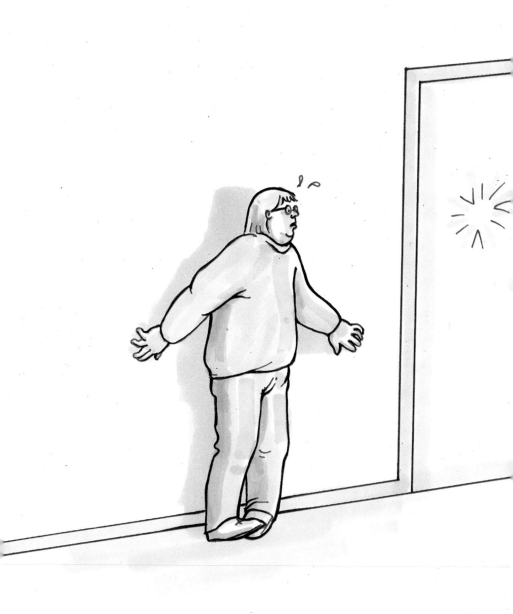

Steve came in and
saw the mess.

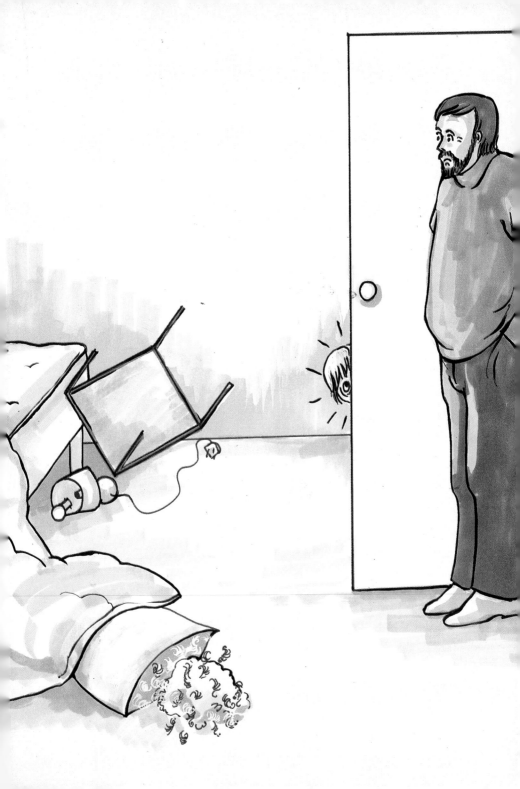

He found Bob hiding
behind the door.

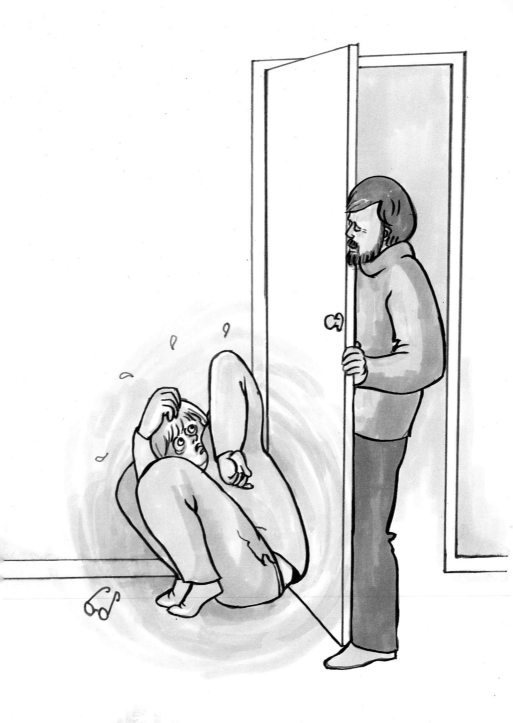

"Don't be afraid," said Steve.
"I'm not going to hurt you."

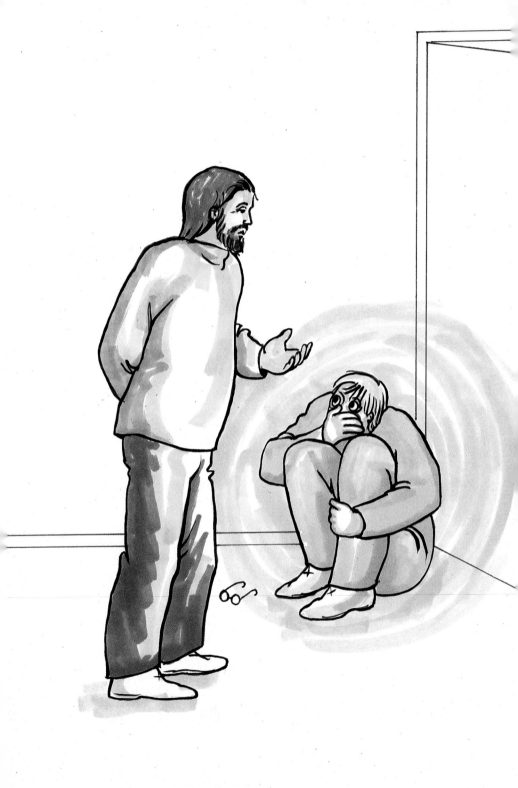

"What's the matter?"
asked Steve.
"It's a secret," said Bob.

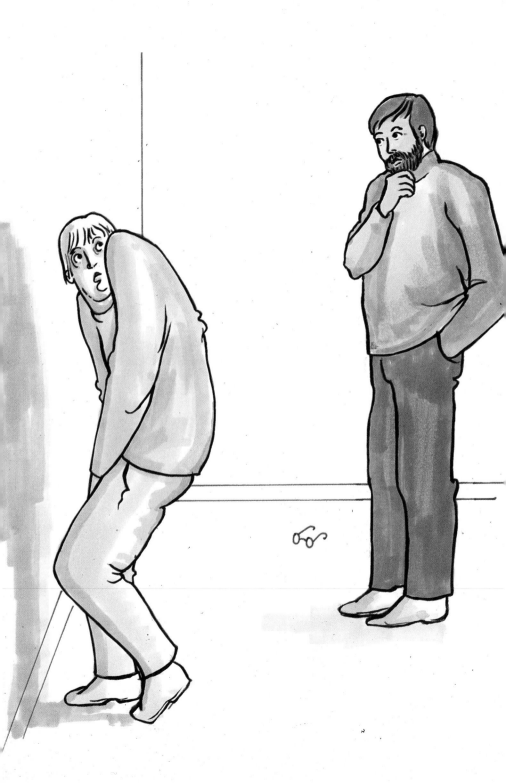

Bob clutched his trousers.
Steve said, "Your trousers
are private. Did you think
I was going to touch them?"

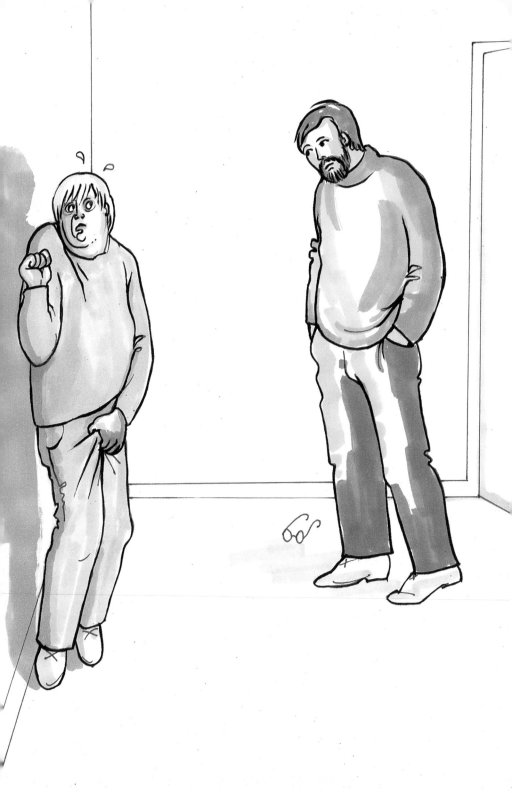

"Yes!" shouted Bob.

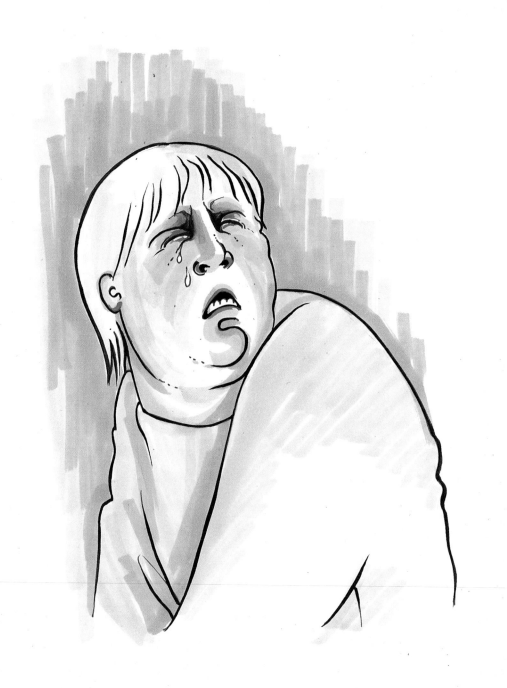

"Has someone hurt
your bottom?" asked Steve.

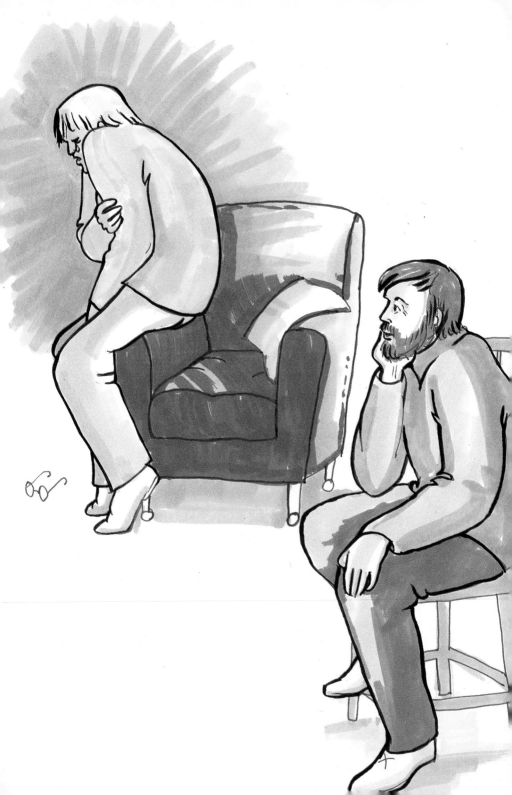

"He used to come in at night,
and do things to my bum,"
said Bob.
"It hurt, and I didn't like it.
He told me not to tell."

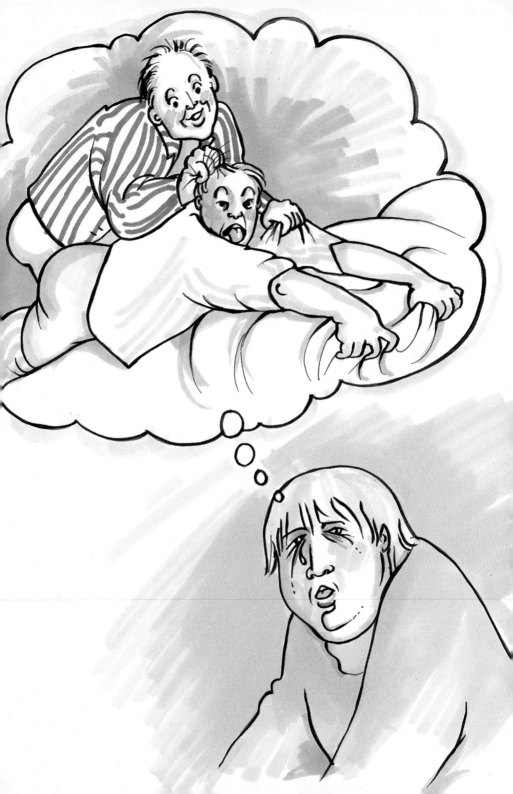

Steve listened carefully.
"That's terrible," he said.

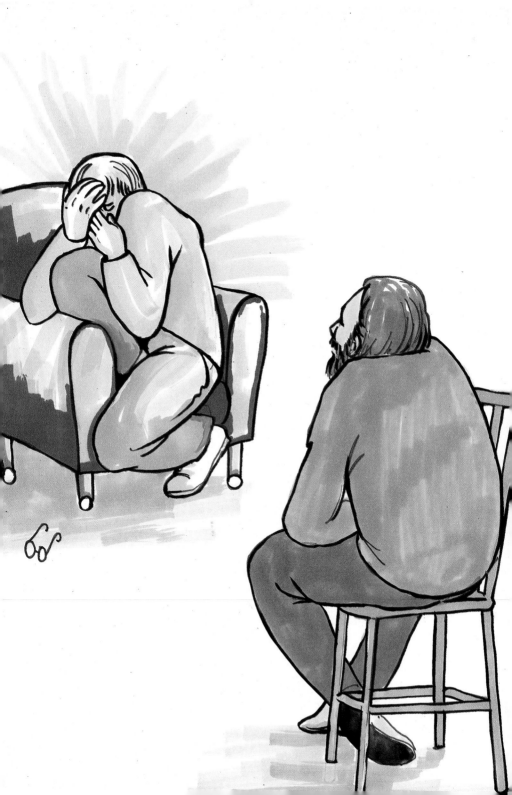

Bob told Steve lots of things.

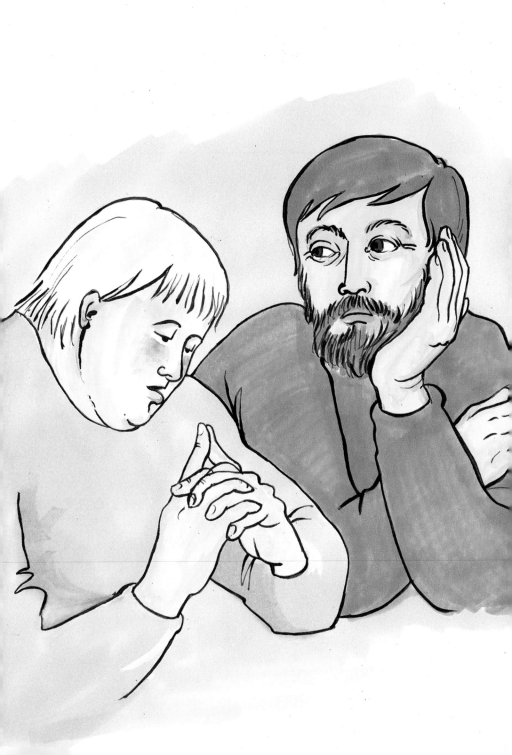

Jon knocked on the door.
"Is Bob alright?" he asked.

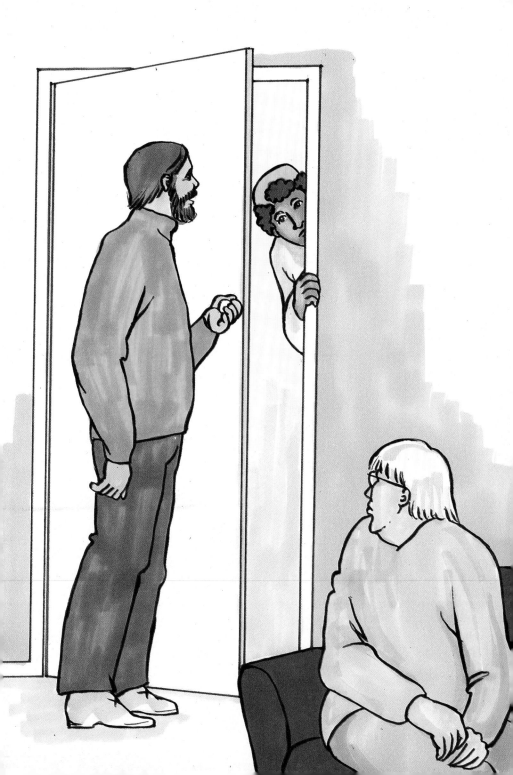

"Bob has been hurt," said Steve.
"He had a horrid time
where he used to live."

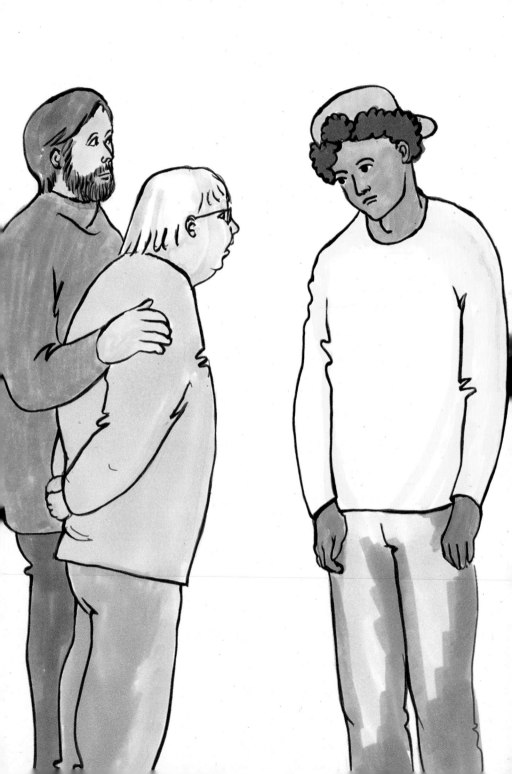

"I'm sorry I frightened you,"
said Bob.
"That's alright," said Jon.

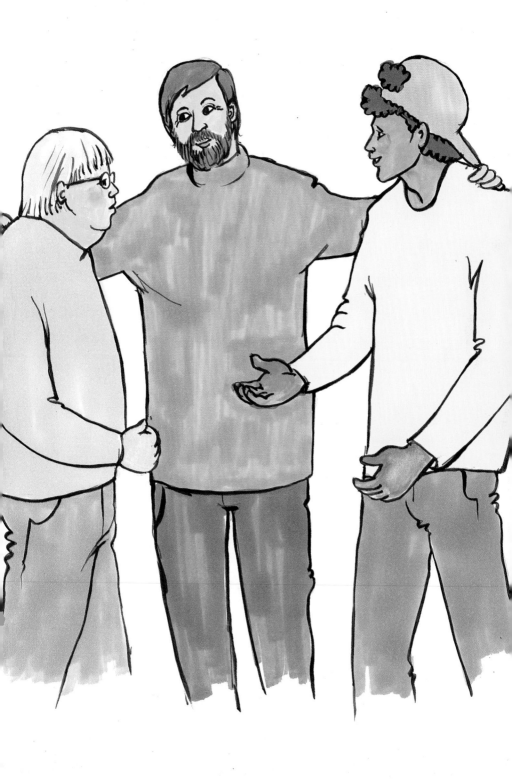

Everyone helped Bob clear up.

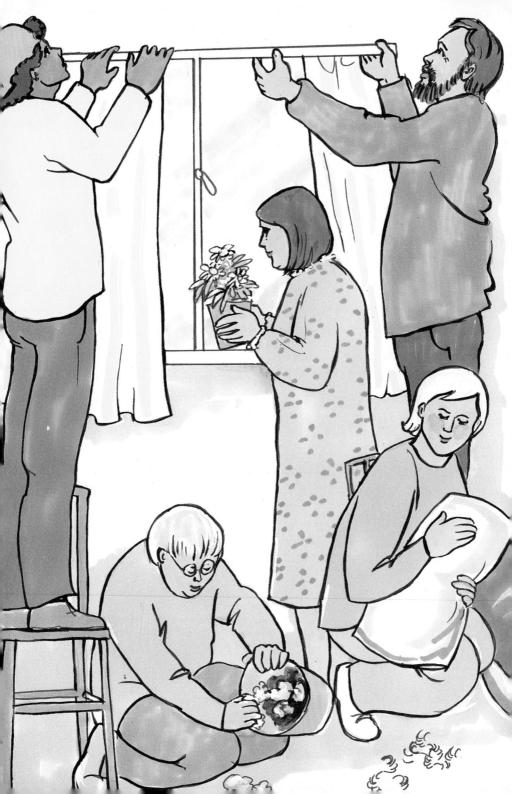

At last everyone could relax.
Steve said they had lots
more talking to do.

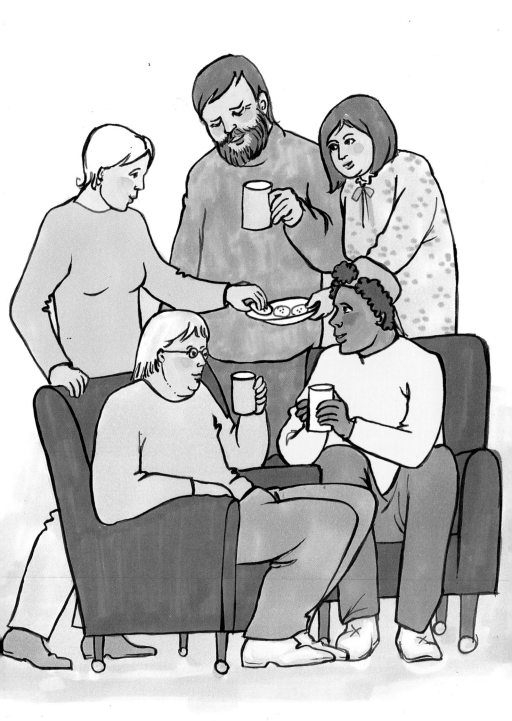

Books in the Sovereign Series:

WHEN MUM DIED / WHEN DAD DIED*
This pair of full colour picture books have a gentle but honest and straightforward approach to death in the family. In a simple, but moving way, the pictures tell the story of the death of a parent, informing the readers about the facts of death and the feelings of grief.

PETER'S NEW HOME / A NEW HOME IN THE COMMUNITY
For people with learning disabilities moving home can be a frightening experience. Proper preparation is vital for a happy transition.
In **Peter's New Home,** Peter leaves his family to go to a group home.
A New Home in the Community tells how Simon leaves a hospital where he has lived for many years.

JENNY SPEAKS OUT* / BOB TELLS ALL*
These books are designed to enable a person with learning disabilities to open up about their experience of sexual abuse.

In preparation:
HUGGING AND TOUCHING
Janet wants someone to hug her but always picks the wrong person. This story tells how she learns when she can and can't hug or touch people.

Other books by the same authors:

Sinason, V., *Mental Handicap and the Human Condition. New Approaches from the Tavistock.* London, Free Association Books, 1992.
Hollins, S., & Grimer, M., *Going Somewhere: People with Mental Handicaps and their Pastoral Care.* New Library of Pastoral Care. London, SPCK, 1988.
Craft, M., Bicknell, J., & Hollins, S., (eds.), *Mental Handicap; A Multidisciplinary Approach.* London, Bailliere Tyndell, 1985.

BEYOND WORDS
counselling people with learning disabilities

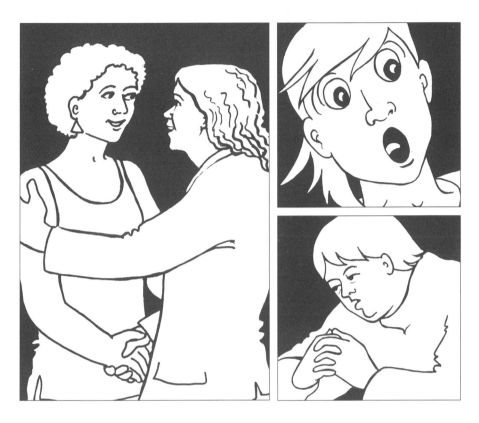

Editor: Professor Sheila Hollins

Illustrations and Design: Beth Webb

These beautiful books from St. George's Mental Health Library explain the difficult things of life to adults with learning disabilities. They also help carers to talk about sensitive topics. The books communicate powerfully but gently, through colour, mime and symbol providing an effective and invaluable counselling tool.

BOOKS BEYOND WORDS have been carefully designed to support the emotional development and counselling of people with learning disabilities.

The books deal with subjects that the Series Editor, a Professor of Psychiatry of Learning Disability, and her co-authors, who are Senior Practitioners have found to be crucial: for example, disability, dependency, sexuality and mortality.

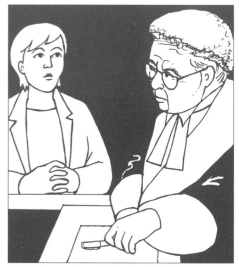

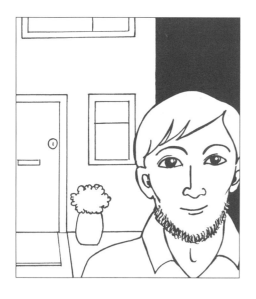

These full colour picture books provide an effective and invaluable counselling tool, assisting people to adjust to change, to accept themselves, to enable them to have satisfying relationships and to make their own decisions.

They also help carers in finding a way to deal with sensitive topics. The books also offer the 'reader' a positive direction and reassurance for the future. People with learning disabilities enjoy owning their own copies.

Books Beyond Words utilise special techniques of non-verbal communication, blending emotionally keyed colours, body language, mime and symbols. The effect of this is to speak clearly to the 'reader', explaining difficult and painful experiences with 'language beyond words'.

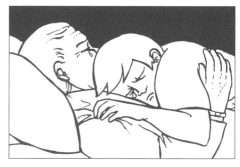

Books in Print

Each of the following books is one of a pair in which the same theme is explored with different people or in a different setting.

Jenny Speaks Out (1992) / Bob Tells All (1993)

Sheila Hollins and Valerie Sinason.
Shortlisted for Book Trust and Joseph Rowntree Foundation 1994 Read Easy Awards.
These books are designed to enable a person with learning disabilities to open up about their experience of sexual abuse.

*Hug Me – Touch Me (1994) / Making Friends (1995)

Sheila Hollins and Terry Roth.
* Winner of the Book Trust and Joseph Rowntree Foundation 1994 Read Easy Awards in the best author category.
Janet (in Hug Me – Touch Me) and Neil (in Making Friends) want someone to hug, but they always pick the wrong person. These two books tell the story of how each learns when they can and can't hug or touch.

When Mum Died / When Dad Died 2nd edition (1994)

Sheila Hollins and Lester Sireling.
Shortlisted for Book Trust and Joseph Rowntree Foundation 1990 Read Easy Awards (1st edition).
Each of these two books tells the story of the death of a parent. Gently and straightforwardly, the events of death are presented and the feelings of grief are experienced.

Peter's New Home / A New Home in the Community (1993)

Sheila Hollins and Deborah Hutchinson.
Shortlisted for Book Trust and Joseph Rowntree Foundation 1994 Read Easy Awards.
For people with learning disabilities moving home can be a frightening experience. Proper preparation is vital for a happy transition. In Peter's New Home, Peter leaves his family to go to a group home. A New Home in the Community tells how Simon leaves a hospital where he has lived for many years.

continued over

Going To Court (1994)

Sheila Hollins with Valerie Sinason and Julie Boniface.
This book is about a victim who is helped to be a witness in a Crown Court.
The pictures are designed to fit any crime and any verdict.

You're Under Arrest (1996)

Sheila Hollins with Isabel Clare and Glynis Murphy.
What happens if you are accused of a crime? This book takes the accused step by step through the police procedures.

You're On Trial (1996)

Sheila Hollins with Glynis Murphy and Isabel Clare.
This book continues the story of You're Nicked, from being charged to becoming a defendant in a Magistrates' Court. It introduces all those involved and offers a range of alternative outcomes.

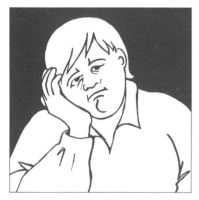

Feeling Blue (1995)

Sheila Hollins and Jenny Curran.
Ron loses interest in eating, swimming and other activities he usually enjoys. He becomes irritable and withdrawn. Feeling blue shows what happens to Ron when he is depressed, and how he is helped to feel better.

BEYOND WORDS
counselling people with learning disabilities

Order form available from
Mrs Freda Macey, Department of Psychiatry of Disability,
St. George's Hospital Medical School, Cranmer Terrace, London SW17 ORE, UK.
TEL: 0181 725 5501 FAX: 0181 672 1070 e. mail: s.hollins@sghms.ac.uk.

ORDER FORM:

Name ....

Address ....

....

....Telephone ....

Please send	No. of copies	Cost
When Dad Died 2nd edition	....	£ ....
When Mum Died 2nd edition	....	£ ....
Jenny Speaks Out	....	£ ....
Jenny Speaks Out looseleaf version	....	£ ....
Bob Tells All	....	£ ....
Bob Tells All looseleaf version	....	£ ....
Peter's New Home	....	£ ....
A New Home in the Community	....	£ ....
Hug Me – Touch Me	....	£ ....
Making Friends	....	£ ....
Going to Court	....	£ ....
You're Under Arrest	....	£ ....
You're On Trial	....	£ ....
Feeling Blue	....	£ ....
Going to the Doctor	....	£ ....

TOTAL £ ....

For a free copy of guidance notes on the use of books please tick ❏
For a free copy of looseleaf French/German* translation please tick ❏

*Delete as appropriate   **FOR PRICES — SEE OVER**

BEYOND WORDS
counselling people with learning disabilities

St. George's Mental Health Library:
The Sovereign Series

List of Titles

For orders please complete the form overleaf.
UK prices: books and laminated looseleaf £10.00 each.
Overseas prices: £12.50 each *(sterling cheques drawn on UK bank only please)*.
All prices include postage and packing. Prices correct at time of printing.

When Dad Died	*Jenny Speaks Out*
When Mum Died	*Looseleaf version*
Peter's New Home	*Bob Tells All*
A Home in the Community	*Looseleaf version*
Hug Me – Touch Me	*Going to Court*
Making Friends	*You're Under Arrest*
	You're On Trial
Feeling Blue	*Going to the Doctor*

PLEASE SEND YOUR ORDER WITH PAYMENT TO:

Mrs Freda Macey
Department of Psychiatry of Disability
St. George's Hospital Medical School
Cranmer Terrace, London
SW17 ORE, UK.

TEL: 0181 725 5501
FAX: 0181 672 1070
e. mail: s.hollins@sghms.ac.uk

FOR ORDER FORM — SEE OVER

St. George's Mental Health Library :The Sovereign Series
ORDER FORM : Photocopy as needed

Please print

Your name ....

Your address ....

....

....

Telephone ....

The books are all £7.50 each including post and packaging (UK); £8.50 for overseas orders. Price correct at time of printing. A small number of sets of laminated looseleaf versions of the books marked * are available at a price of £15.00 on request.
Please send me:

( ) copies of When Dad Died*   £.......
( ) copies of looseleaf version   £.......
( ) copies of When Mum Died   £.......
( ) copies of Jenny Speaks Out*   £.......
( ) copies of looseleaf version   £.......
( ) copies of Bob Tells All*   £.......
( ) copies of looseleaf version   £.......
( ) copies of Peter's New Home   £.......
( ) copies of A New Home in the Community   £.......
In preparation:
( ) copies of Hugging and Touching   £.......

TOTAL   £.......

CHEQUES SHOULD BE MADE PAYABLE TO:
ST. GEORGE'S HOSPITAL SPECIAL TRUSTEES

PLEASE SEND YOUR ORDER, WITH PAYMENT TO:
Mrs. Freda Macey, Division of Psychiatry of Disability, Department of Mental Health Sciences, St. George's Hospital Medical School, Cranmer Terrace, London, SW17 0RE, UK.